Overcoming Diabetes

Sending Diabetes Into Remission

GW00771181

Dr. Frederick Boly

Copyright

TABLE OF CONTENT

Introduction

Welcome to "Overcoming Diabetes," a comprehensive guide designed to empower individuals on their journey to manage and conquer diabetes. In this book, we explore the intricacies of diabetes, from understanding its various types to offering practical insights into effective lifestyle adjustments. Discover strategies to navigate blood sugar spikes and lows, delve into medication options, and build a robust support system. Uncover the importance of monitoring blood sugar levels and learn about natural remedies for holistic well-being. Additionally, find valuable tips for achieving diabetes remission and preventing setbacks. Join us on this empowering expedition towards a healthier and more fulfilling life with diabetes.

Understanding Diabetes

Understanding diabetes is crucial for anyone newly diagnosed and those seeking comprehensive insights into this condition. Diabetes is a metabolic disorder characterized by elevated blood sugar levels, often caused by the body's inability to produce or effectively use insulin. Insulin is a hormone that regulates sugar absorption into cells for energy.

There are two main types of diabetes: Type 1 and Type 2. Type 1 diabetes occurs when the immune system mistakenly attacks and destroys insulin-producing cells in the pancreas. It's commonly diagnosed in children and young adults. On the other hand, Type 2 diabetes usually develops later in life when the body becomes resistant to insulin or doesn't produce enough.

Risk factors for diabetes include genetics, lifestyle, and environmental factors. Family history, obesity, unhealthy eating habits, and physical inactivity can contribute to its development. Understanding these factors helps individuals make informed choices to reduce their risk.

The hallmark symptom of diabetes is elevated blood sugar levels, leading to symptoms like excessive thirst, frequent urination, fatigue, and blurred vision. Early diagnosis is crucial for effective management.

Managing diabetes involves lifestyle adjustments. Healthy eating habits, regular exercise, and stress management play pivotal roles. Monitoring blood sugar levels is essential to track progress and make informed decisions. This involves regularly checking blood sugar using a glucose meter and interpreting the results.

For those with Type 1 diabetes, insulin therapy is often necessary. In Type 2 diabetes, medications, lifestyle changes, and sometimes insulin may be prescribed. It's important to work closely with healthcare professionals to determine the most effective treatment plan.

In conclusion, understanding diabetes is foundational for navigating its complexities. Recognizing the causes, types, and symptoms empowers individuals to take charge of their health. With proactive management, lifestyle adjustments, and ongoing support, those affected can lead fulfilling lives while effectively managing their diabetes.

Complications and Other Diseases Linked to Diabetes

Diabetes, if not properly managed, can lead to various complications and contribute to the development of other diseases. It's essential to be aware of these potential risks to prioritize preventive measures and comprehensive healthcare.

1. Cardiovascular Diseases: Diabetes significantly increases the risk of heart diseases and strokes. High blood sugar levels can damage blood vessels, leading to atherosclerosis and increasing the likelihood of heart attacks and strokes.

2. Kidney Disease (Nephropathy): Diabetes is a leading cause of kidney disease. Persistent high blood sugar levels can damage the kidneys over time, impairing their ability to filter waste from the blood.

3. Eye Complications (Retinopathy): Prolonged diabetes can cause damage to the blood vessels in the eyes, leading to diabetic retinopathy. This condition can result in vision impairment and, if left untreated, may lead to blindness.

4. Nerve Damage (Neuropathy): Diabetes can cause nerve damage, resulting in neuropathy. This condition often affects the feet and legs, causing pain, tingling, and numbness. Severe neuropathy can lead to infections and, in some cases, amputations.

5. Peripheral Vascular Disease: Diabetes can impair blood circulation, especially in the lower extremities, leading to peripheral vascular disease. This condition increases the risk of infections, slow healing, and potential amputations.

6. Skin Conditions: Diabetes may contribute to skin problems, including bacterial and fungal infections. High blood sugar levels create an environment conducive to skin issues, necessitating careful hygiene and skincare.

7. Altered Immune Function: Diabetes can weaken the immune system, making individuals more susceptible to infections. It can also hinder the body's ability to heal, increasing the severity of wounds and infections.

8. Increased Risk of Other Conditions: Diabetes is associated with an increased risk of conditions like high blood pressure and high cholesterol. These factors further elevate the risk of cardiovascular diseases.

Understanding these potential complications underscores the importance of proactive diabetes management. Regular medical check-ups, adherence to prescribed treatments, lifestyle modifications, and maintaining a healthy weight are key components in preventing or managing these diabetes-related complications. By addressing these aspects, individuals with diabetes can strive for better overall health and well-being.

Coping with a New Diagnosis

A diabetes diagnosis can be overwhelming, but with the right strategies, individuals can navigate this new chapter and effectively cope with the challenges that come with managing the condition.

1. Emotional Support: It's normal to experience a range of emotions such as shock, fear, or even

denial. Seek emotional support from friends, family, or support groups. Sharing your feelings can provide comfort and reassurance.

2. Educate Yourself: Knowledge is empowering. Take the time to learn about diabetes, its causes, and how it affects the body. Understanding the condition is a crucial step in managing it effectively.

3. Build a Healthcare Team: Establish a strong relationship with healthcare professionals, including doctors, diabetes educators, and dietitians. They can provide guidance, answer questions, and help you create a personalized management plan.

4. Healthy Lifestyle Choices: Adopting a healthy lifestyle is key to managing diabetes. Focus on balanced nutrition, regular exercise, and sufficient sleep. Small, sustainable changes can have a significant impact on overall well-being.

5. Set Realistic Goals: Break down the management process into achievable goals. Whether it's maintaining a certain blood sugar level or incorporating daily physical activity, setting realistic objectives fosters a sense of accomplishment.

6. Monitor Blood Sugar Levels: Regularly monitoring blood sugar levels is essential. This provides valuable insights into how lifestyle choices and medications impact your body, allowing for better-informed decisions.

7. Connect with Others: Joining diabetes support groups or online communities can provide a sense of camaraderie. Sharing experiences, tips, and strategies with others who understand what you're going through can be immensely beneficial.

8. Communicate with Loved Ones: Educate your close circle about diabetes, its challenges, and how they can support you. Open communication fosters understanding and ensures you have a reliable support system.

9. Stay Positive: Maintaining a positive mindset is crucial. Focus on the aspects of life you can control, celebrate achievements, and recognize that managing diabetes is a continuous journey.

10. Professional Counseling: If the emotional burden becomes overwhelming, consider seeking professional counseling or therapy. A mental health

professional can provide guidance and support tailored to your emotional needs.

Coping with a new diabetes diagnosis involves a combination of education, support, and self-care. By embracing these strategies and building a solid foundation for diabetes management, individuals can lead fulfilling lives while effectively addressing the challenges posed by the condition.

Importance of Early Management

Early management of diabetes is like planting a seed for a healthy future. When diabetes is detected early, it allows us to take quick and smart actions to keep our bodies in balance.

Imagine it as a superhero move – catching the villain (high blood sugar) before it causes trouble. Early on, diabetes might not show big signs, but it's secretly affecting our body. Taking action early means we can stop these sneak attacks.

Early management helps prevent complications, like problems with our heart, kidneys, and eyes. It's like building a strong fortress to protect our body against potential harm.

Think of it this way – the sooner we start taking care of diabetes, the better our chances of living a happy and healthy life. It's our way of saying, "Not today, diabetes!" So, don't wait. Act early, be a superhero for your health!

Understanding Diabetes Remission

Understanding diabetes remission is like witnessing a positive transformation in your health journey. Diabetes remission refers to a state where blood sugar levels return to normal without the need for diabetes medications or interventions. It's akin to a temporary pause in the condition's active presence.

This achievement is often associated with substantial lifestyle changes, including adopting a healthy diet, engaging in regular physical activity, and achieving weight loss. During diabetes remission, the body's ability to regulate blood sugar improves, offering a break from the constant management associated with diabetes.

It's important to note that diabetes remission doesn't imply a permanent cure. Maintaining the lifestyle changes that led to remission is crucial, as diabetes can return if healthy habits are not sustained. Regular monitoring, healthcare guidance, and ongoing commitment to a healthy lifestyle are key elements in understanding and achieving diabetes remission.
Withy the guidelines from this book I am confident you will be able to send your diabetes into remission. Let's get started !

Chapter 1

The Basics of Diabetes

Types of Diabetes

Understanding the different types of diabetes is like knowing the characters in a story – each with its own traits and challenges. There are primarily two main types: Type 1 and Type 2.

1. Type 1 Diabetes:
   - The Body's Mix-Up: In Type 1, it's like the body's defense system goes haywire. The immune system mistakenly attacks and destroys the "insulin factories" in the pancreas.
   - Common Heroes: Often starts in childhood or early adulthood. People with Type 1 need insulin to survive because their bodies can't produce it.

2. Type 2 Diabetes:
   - The Resistance Story: In Type 2, the body resists the superhero insulin or doesn't make

enough of it. This means the sugar can't get into the cells properly.

- Late Arrival: Typically shows up in adults, but nowadays, even some youngsters are facing it. It's often linked to lifestyle factors like unhealthy eating and lack of exercise.

3. Gestational Diabetes:

- Temporary Twist: Sometimes, there's a special episode during pregnancy called gestational diabetes. It usually goes away after the baby is born, but it's essential to manage during pregnancy for a healthy mom and baby.

Understanding these diabetes types is like having a map for the journey. Each type needs a different approach, but with the right knowledge and support, people can navigate their way to better health. It's like knowing the characters in the diabetes story – each one needing its own kind of attention and care.

How Insulin Works

Imagine insulin as the key that unlocks the doors for sugar to enter your body's cells. It's like a friendly messenger ensuring that the energy from sugar gets inside and is used properly. Let's dive into the details of how this process works in simple terms.

1. Sugar and the Energy Game:
- Our bodies break down the food we eat into sugar, known as glucose.
- Glucose is like the superhero fuel that gives us energy to move, think, and do everything.

2. The Cell Door Locks:
- Cells are like tiny houses in our body, and they need glucose for energy.
- But, cells have locked doors, and glucose can't just walk in by itself.

3. Insulin, the Master Key:
- Now enters insulin – the magical key that unlocks the doors of cells.
- When we eat, the pancreas (an organ in our belly) releases insulin into the bloodstream.

4. The Glucose Journey:
- Insulin helps glucose leave the bloodstream and enter the cells.
- It's like a helpful guide directing glucose to the right places.

5. Balancing Act:

- Insulin doesn't just let all the glucose in at once. It's like a smart manager, making sure the right amount enters so that everything stays in balance.

6. Storage Mode:

- Sometimes, when there's extra glucose, insulin helps store it in the liver for later use. It's like saving some energy for a rainy day.

7. Insulin's Break Time:

- After insulin does its job, it takes a break. The insulin levels drop until it's needed again.

Understanding how insulin works is like knowing the conductor in an orchestra – it ensures that every part of the body gets the energy it needs at the right time. When this process goes smoothly, our body functions like a well-oiled machine. However, in diabetes, this harmony is disrupted, and insulin might not work as effectively. That's when managing insulin becomes crucial to maintain the delicate balance of energy in our bodies.

Blood Sugar Monitoring

Blood sugar monitoring is like keeping an eye on the fuel gauge in your car – it helps you know if everything is running smoothly or if there's a need for adjustments. It's a crucial part of managing diabetes, ensuring that your sugar levels stay in the right range for a healthy and balanced life.

How to Do It:
Monitoring blood sugar involves a small device called a glucose meter and a tiny drop of blood. Here's how it works:

1. Preparation: Wash your hands to make sure they're clean. Clean the spot where you'll get the drop of blood, usually a fingertip.

2. Pricking the Finger: Use a small device called a lancet to gently prick your fingertip. It might feel like a tiny pinch.

3. Collecting the Drop: Let a small drop of blood form, and carefully place it on a test strip. The test strip goes into the glucose meter.

4. The Glucose Meter Magic: The meter quickly measures the amount of sugar in your blood and shows the result on its screen.

5. Recording the Numbers: Keep a record of your readings. It's like creating a blood sugar diary that helps you and your healthcare team understand how your body responds to different foods and activities.

Correct Ways to Do It:
To ensure accurate readings, follow these tips:

1. Regular Schedule: Check your blood sugar at the times recommended by your healthcare team – usually before meals, sometimes after meals, and maybe before bedtime.

2. Proper Storage: Store your test strips and glucose meter as instructed. Extreme temperatures can affect accuracy.

3. Calibration Check: Make sure your meter is calibrated correctly. Some meters need occasional checks to ensure they're giving accurate readings.

4. Clean Equipment: Keep your meter and lancet device clean. Regular cleaning helps maintain accuracy and prevents infections.

5. Proper Technique: Follow the instructions provided with your glucose meter. Using the correct technique ensures reliable results.

Importance of Blood Sugar Monitoring:

1. Control and Adjustments: Monitoring allows you to see how your body responds to food, exercise, and medications. If your sugar levels are too high or too low, you can make necessary adjustments to keep them in check.

2. Early Detection: Regular monitoring helps catch fluctuations early, preventing potential complications. It's like having an early warning system for your health.

3. Informed Decision-Making: Understanding your blood sugar levels empowers you to make informed decisions about your lifestyle and treatment plan. It's like having a map to guide you on your journey to better health.

4. Communication with Healthcare Team: Sharing your blood sugar readings with your healthcare team helps them tailor your diabetes management plan to your specific needs. It's like working together on a personalized strategy for your well-being.

In summary, blood sugar monitoring is a practical and essential tool for managing diabetes. It's not just about numbers; it's about understanding your body, making informed choices, and taking control of your health journey.

Chapter 2

Lifestyle Adjustments- Healthy Eating Habits

Welcome to Chapter 2: Lifestyle Adjustments – Healthy Eating where we embark on a journey of cultivating healthy habits, starting with nourishing our bodies through smart and enjoyable eating. This chapter is your guide to adopting balanced and sustainable eating habits that harmonize with managing diabetes. Together, we'll explore the flavors of nutritious choices and discover how they contribute to a fulfilling and healthful lifestyle. Get ready to embrace the joy of wholesome eating, making it a cornerstone in your quest for wellness and balance with diabetes. Let's savor the path to nourishment and vitality.

Understanding Nutritional Basics

Understanding the nutritional basics is like having a compass that guides us in making healthy choices for our bodies. Let's break down the key elements – macronutrients, micronutrients, and fiber – in simple terms.

Macronutrients:

Think of macronutrients as the big players in the food game. There are three main types:
1. Carbohydrates: These are like the body's preferred energy source, found in foods like bread, rice, and fruits.
2. Proteins: Proteins are like the building blocks for our bodies. They help repair tissues and can be found in meats, beans, and nuts.
3. Fats: Fats are like the energy reserves. They're in oils, butter, and avocados. We need them, but it's about choosing the right kinds in the right amounts.

Micronutrients:
Now, micronutrients are like the tiny superheroes. They may be small, but they play essential roles:

1. Vitamins: Imagine them as mini-boosters – vitamin C for a strong immune system (found in oranges) and vitamin A for healthy eyes (in carrots).

2. Minerals: These are like the body's helpers –
calcium for strong bones (in dairy) and iron for
healthy blood (in spinach).

Fiber:
Fiber is like the body's janitor – it keeps things clean
and moving smoothly. Found in fruits, vegetables,
and whole grains, fiber helps with digestion and
keeps our gut happy.

Understanding these basics is like having a
superhero team in our food choices. Carbs give us
quick energy, proteins build and repair, fats provide
a backup energy source, vitamins and minerals
ensure our body functions well, and fiber keeps
everything running smoothly.

Making informed food choices is about creating a
balanced team of these nutrients on our plate. It's
not about excluding certain foods but finding the
right mix that supports our body's needs.

In summary, the nutritional basics are the ABCs of
healthy eating. They guide us to choose foods that
fuel and nourish our bodies, ensuring we have the
energy and nutrients needed for a vibrant and active

life. It's like laying the groundwork for a strong and resilient body – a foundation for making smart and informed food choices every day.

Creating a Diabetes-Friendly Plate

Creating a diabetes-friendly plate is like being a chef who carefully chooses the right ingredients to make a delicious and healthy meal. This section is your recipe for balancing different food elements on your plate, ensuring your body gets the right mix to manage blood sugar effectively.

Portion Control:

Imagine your plate as a canvas, and portion control is like deciding how much paint to use. It's about not too much and not too little. Controlling portions helps manage the amount of food you eat, preventing blood sugar from spiking.

Balancing Carbohydrates, Proteins, and Fats:

Picture your plate as a team, and each food group plays a special role:

1. Carbohydrates: They're like the energy providers. Choose whole grains, fruits, and veggies for a steady release of energy.

2. Proteins: Proteins are the builders. Include sources like lean meats, beans, and nuts to help repair and grow your body.

3. Fats: Fats are the backup energy. Pick healthy fats like those in avocados and olive oil. They're essential but need to be in the right amounts.

Constructing Balanced Meals:

Building a balanced plate is like creating a harmonious symphony of flavors. Aim for a mix of colors and textures:

1. Vegetables: Fill half your plate with colorful veggies. They're like the superheroes, packed with nutrients.

2. Proteins: Add a palm-sized portion of lean protein. It's like the hero in your meal, supporting your body.

3. Carbohydrates: Include a fist-sized portion of whole grains or starchy veggies. They're like the sidekick, providing energy.

4. Fats: Add a thumb-sized portion of healthy fats. They're like the wise mentor, keeping things in balance.

This approach to your plate is like having a blueprint for a healthy meal that supports your body's needs and keeps blood sugar levels in check. It's not about restricting foods but about making thoughtful choices that work together.

Smart Food Choices for Diabetes Management

Creating smart food choices for diabetes management is akin to assembling a nutritional toolkit that empowers your body. Let's embark on this journey, understanding foods to avoid and the delightful options that contribute to a diabetes-friendly meal.

Foods to Avoid:

1. Sugary Beverages:

- The Culprit: Regular sodas, fruit juices, and sweetened drinks.
- Why to Avoid: These sugary concoctions swiftly elevate blood sugar levels, contributing to unstable glucose levels.

2. Processed Snacks:
- The Culprit: Packaged chips, cookies, and processed snacks.
- Why to Avoid: Laden with unhealthy fats, excessive salt, and refined carbs, these snacks can disrupt blood sugar control.

3. White Flour Products:
- The Culprit: White bread, white rice, and refined flour products.
- Why to Avoid: These rapidly digestible carbs can lead to rapid spikes in blood sugar, akin to a quick burst of energy followed by a crash.

4. High-Sugar Cereals:
- The Culprit: Sugary breakfast cereals.
- Why to Avoid: These seemingly innocent bowls can be loaded with hidden sugars, affecting blood sugar levels throughout the day.

5. Sweetened Yogurts:

- The Culprit: Flavored yogurts with added sugars.
- Why to Avoid: While yogurt itself can be a healthy choice, added sugars in flavored varieties can turn this into a sugary trap.

6. Candy and Sweets:
  - The Culprit: Candies, chocolates, and sugary treats.
  - Why to Avoid: These delightful indulgences can cause rapid spikes in blood sugar, demanding cautious consumption.

7. Fried Foods:
  - The Culprit: Deep-fried delights like fries and fried chicken.
  - Why to Avoid: Fried foods are often high in unhealthy fats, contributing to weight gain and insulin resistance.

8. Excessive Alcohol:
  - The Culprit: Overindulgence in alcoholic beverages.
  - Why to Avoid: Alcohol can lead to fluctuations in blood sugar levels, especially when consumed without food, posing challenges for diabetes management.

Foods to Embrace:

1. Colorful Vegetables:
   - The Hero: Broccoli, spinach, bell peppers, and colorful veggies.
   - How They Help: Rich in fiber, vitamins, and antioxidants, vegetables stabilize blood sugar and promote overall health.

2. Lean Proteins:
   - The Hero: Chicken, turkey, fish, tofu, and legumes.
   - How They Help: Proteins aid in muscle maintenance, induce a feeling of fullness, and don't cause significant blood sugar spikes.

3. Healthy Fats:
   - The Hero: Avocados, nuts, seeds, and olive oil.
   - How They Help: Providing essential fatty acids, healthy fats contribute to satiety and support overall well-being.

4. Whole Grains:
   - The Hero: Quinoa, brown rice, oats, and whole wheat.
   - How They Help: Whole grains release energy gradually, preventing sudden spikes in blood sugar.

5. Berries:
   - The Hero: Blueberries, strawberries, and raspberries.
   - How They Help: Packed with fiber and antioxidants, berries offer a sweet fix without causing significant blood sugar swings.

6. Greek Yogurt:
   - The Hero: Unsweetened Greek yogurt.
   - How It Helps: A protein-rich and low-sugar alternative, supporting digestion and blood sugar control.

7. Leafy Greens:
   - The Hero: Kale, spinach, and Swiss chard.
   - How They Help: Low in carbs and rich in nutrients, leafy greens contribute to a diabetes-friendly plate.

8. Legumes:
   - The Hero: Lentils, chickpeas, and black beans.
   - How They Help: High in fiber and protein, legumes offer a gradual release of energy, promoting stable blood sugar levels.

Constructing a Diabetes-Friendly Plate:

33

Building a balanced plate involves a mindful combination of these heroes:
1. Vegetables: Fill half your plate with colorful vegetables.
2. Proteins: Include a palm-sized portion of lean protein.
3. Healthy Carbs: Add a fist-sized portion of whole grains or starchy vegetables.
4. Healthy Fats: Integrate a thumb-sized portion of healthy fats.

Hydration Matters:
Water is the unsung hero in diabetes management. Staying hydrated helps regulate blood sugar and supports overall health.

In conclusion, navigating a diabetes-friendly meal involves making thoughtful choices that prioritize nutrient-rich options while avoiding pitfalls laden with sugars and unhealthy fats. It's about curating a palette of foods that not only satiate your taste buds but also contribute to stable blood sugar levels and overall well-being. Remember, these choices aren't restrictions but steps towards a vibrant and healthful lifestyle.

Meal Planning Strategies

Meal planning strategies are like having a roadmap for delicious and healthful eating. Let's break down this section into bite-sized pieces, making it easy to understand.

Meal Prepping:
Imagine spending a little time upfront to prepare your meals for the week. It's like having ready-to-go meals that fit your health goals. Chop veggies, cook grains, and portion proteins – it's a time-saver when life gets busy.

Creating Grocery Lists:
Think of grocery lists as your shopping sidekick. Jot down what you need for the week, ensuring you have all the ingredients for balanced and nutritious meals. It's like ensuring you have all the puzzle pieces before starting to play.

Adapting Recipes:
Recipes are like guidelines, not strict rules. Adapt them to suit your taste and health needs. Swap ingredients for healthier options – it's like giving your favorite dish a nutritious makeover.

Practical Tools:
Utilize tools like measuring cups and a food scale. They're like the handy assistants in your kitchen, ensuring portion control and balanced meals. These tools make it easier to keep track of what you're eating.

Incorporating Healthy Eating:
Healthy eating isn't about drastic changes; it's about small, sustainable shifts. Include a variety of colors and nutrients in your meals. It's like creating a vibrant palette on your plate that supports your well-being.

Everyday Life:
Meal planning isn't a rigid task; it fits into your daily routine. Whether you're a busy professional or a parent on the go, these strategies are adaptable. It's like weaving healthy eating seamlessly into your everyday life.

In essence, meal planning strategies are your allies in creating a balanced and practical approach to eating well. They're like the tools in your toolkit, making it easier to enjoy delicious, nutritious meals without the stress of figuring it out every day.

Building Long-Term Healthy

Building long-term healthy habits is like cultivating a garden for your well-being. Let's explore this section in a few simple steps.

Celebrating Progress:
Think of small victories as stepping stones. Celebrate them! It's like cheering for yourself when you choose a nutritious snack or add a few extra steps to your day. These celebrations build a positive mindset.

Overcoming Challenges:
Challenges are part of the journey, not roadblocks. It's like finding alternative routes when there's construction. Adapt and keep moving forward. Facing challenges is an opportunity to learn and grow.

Integrating Exercise:
Exercise isn't just about hitting the gym; it's any movement that brings you joy. It's like dancing in the living room, taking a stroll, or playing a favorite

sport. Find what you love, and it won't feel like a task.

Sustaining Healthy Habits:
Long-term well-being is about consistency, not perfection. It's like choosing nourishing foods regularly and making movement a part of your routine. These habits become second nature, woven into your lifestyle.

Importance of Routine
Creating a routine is like having a roadmap for your day. It adds structure and makes healthy choices more automatic. It's not about rigid schedules but creating a flow that supports your health goals.

Mindful Choices:
Being mindful is like having a compass for decision-making. Pause, reflect, and make choices aligned with your well-being. It's not about restriction but about making conscious decisions that honor your health.

In summary, building long-term healthy habits is a journey of small victories, adapting to challenges, finding joy in movement, and weaving well-being into your daily life. It's a marathon, not a sprint – a sustainable path toward a healthier and happier you.

Chapter 3

Lifestyle Adjustments- Regular Exercise

Welcome to Chapter 3: Lifestyle Adjustments – Regular Exercise where we explore the vital role of regular exercise in achieving holistic well-being. In this chapter, we unravel the importance of incorporating physical activity into your routine. From boosting energy levels to enhancing mental well-being, discover how exercise becomes a cornerstone in your journey towards a healthier and more vibrant lifestyle. Get ready to lace up your sneakers and embark on a path that not only nurtures your body but also uplifts your spirit. Let's dive into the transformative power of regular exercise for a life filled with vitality and balance.

Understanding the Benefits of Exercise for Diabetics

Role of Exercise in Diabetes Management: Insulin Sensitivity, Blood Glucose Levels, and Blood Sugar Control

Insulin Sensitivity:

Exercise acts like a superhero for insulin sensitivity. Picture insulin as a key, unlocking cells to let glucose in for energy. In diabetes, this key might not work as smoothly. However, when we exercise, especially with activities like walking or dancing, our muscles become more responsive. They start using glucose for energy, even without a lot of assistance from insulin. It's like exercise trains our cells to better understand and work with insulin, making the whole process more efficient.

Managing Blood Glucose Levels:

Exercise is a powerful ally in keeping blood glucose levels in check. When we move our bodies, it signals our muscles to absorb glucose from the blood, acting like a natural blood sugar regulator.

This process happens even without a lot of help from insulin. Imagine exercise as a friendly assistant ensuring that glucose gets used for energy, preventing it from lingering too much in the bloodstream. Regular physical activity not only makes our muscles better at this but also helps lower overall blood sugar levels.

Improving Blood Sugar Control:

Exercise becomes a key player in the daily fight against high blood sugar. By enhancing insulin sensitivity and aiding glucose absorption, exercise actively contributes to better blood sugar control. It's like a routine maintenance task for the body – the more we move, the more efficiently our system manages glucose. This consistent effort, over time, leads to more stable blood sugar levels, reducing the risk of spikes and creating a healthier balance. In essence, exercise is a cornerstone in the comprehensive strategy for managing diabetes, playing a vital role in improving insulin sensitivity, regulating blood glucose levels, and achieving better control over overall blood sugar.

Role of Exercise in Diabetes: Cardiovascular Health, Lowering Heart Disease Risk, and Enhancing Circulation

Managing diabetes involves more than watching blood sugar levels; it's a holistic journey, and exercise becomes a crucial companion in promoting cardiovascular health, lowering the risk of heart disease, and enhancing circulation.

1. Cardiovascular Health:

Think of your heart as the engine of your body. Exercise is like a tune-up that keeps this engine running smoothly. In diabetes, there's a higher risk of heart-related issues, making cardiovascular health a top priority. When we engage in activities like walking, jogging, or cycling, our heart pumps more efficiently, strengthening its muscles. This is akin to giving your heart a good workout, making it resilient and better equipped to handle the challenges posed by diabetes.

2. Lowering Heart Disease Risk:

Diabetes and heart disease often go hand in hand. Exercise serves as a shield, protecting against

43

heart-related complications. Regular physical activity helps manage factors that contribute to heart disease, such as high blood pressure and unhealthy cholesterol levels. It's like creating a fortress around your heart. Exercise not only lowers these risk factors but also improves overall heart function, reducing the likelihood of heart-related issues.

3. Enhancing Circulation:

Imagine your blood vessels as the highways that transport essential nutrients and oxygen throughout your body. Diabetes can sometimes affect these highways, causing circulation issues. Exercise is like traffic control, ensuring a smooth flow. When we move, our blood vessels dilate, allowing blood to circulate more freely. This improved circulation delivers oxygen and nutrients efficiently to various body parts. It's akin to opening up the lanes, preventing traffic jams in your blood vessels and reducing the strain on your heart.

How Exercise Works Its Magic:

Now, let's dive deeper into the mechanisms at play:

- Improved Heart Function: Exercise strengthens the heart muscle, enhancing its ability to pump blood. This increased efficiency reduces the workload on the heart, promoting long-term cardiovascular health.

- Blood Pressure Regulation: Exercise helps maintain healthy blood pressure levels. It's like a natural regulator, ensuring that your blood vessels stay open and the pressure remains within a safe range, reducing the risk of complications.

- Cholesterol Management: Diabetes can sometimes lead to imbalances in cholesterol levels. Exercise acts as a cholesterol manager, increasing levels of 'good' cholesterol (HDL) and lowering 'bad' cholesterol (LDL), contributing to a healthier heart profile.

- Blood Sugar Control: While our focus here is on cardiovascular health, it's crucial to mention that exercise also plays a pivotal role in regulating blood sugar levels. This dual action makes it a cornerstone in comprehensive diabetes management.

Types of Exercise Suitable for Diabetic Patients

Aerobic Exercises and Their Benefits for Diabetes

1. Walking:
Walking is a diabetic-friendly superhero, contributing significantly to managing blood sugar levels. It's like a natural insulin booster – as you walk, your muscles use glucose for energy, helping to regulate blood sugar. This low-impact exercise is accessible to most, making it an excellent choice for individuals with diabetes. It not only improves insulin sensitivity but also aids in weight management, another key aspect for diabetes control. Walking regularly, even in short sessions, can be a game-changer, fostering better overall health and glucose regulation.

2. Cycling:
Cycling pedals its way into diabetes management by enhancing insulin sensitivity. As you cycle, your muscles work hard, utilizing glucose for energy, which helps maintain stable blood sugar levels. It's like a blood sugar balancing act on wheels. Additionally, cycling is a joint-friendly exercise,

making it suitable for those with mobility concerns. Regular cycling also contributes to weight control, reducing the risk of insulin resistance. Whether you choose outdoor biking or stationary cycling, it's a delightful way to promote cardiovascular health while keeping diabetes in check.

3. Swimming:

Diving into swimming provides a refreshing splash of benefits for diabetes. This low-impact aerobic exercise engages major muscle groups, promoting efficient glucose utilization. It's like a cool, underwater dance that supports cardiovascular health without putting stress on the joints. Swimming improves insulin sensitivity, making cells more receptive to insulin's signals. The buoyancy of water provides resistance, contributing to muscle strength and overall fitness. For individuals with diabetes, swimming offers a unique combination of cardiovascular and muscular benefits while being gentle on the body.

Strength Training and Flexibility Activities: Enhancing Diabetes Management

1. Building Muscle Mass for Blood Sugar Control:

47

Strength training serves as a powerhouse in diabetes management, contributing to blood sugar control by sculpting stronger muscles. When you engage in strength training, you're like a builder constructing a foundation of muscle mass. These muscles act as efficient glucose users, helping regulate blood sugar levels. As you strengthen them, it's akin to empowering your body with better tools for managing glucose, a key aspect in diabetes control.

2. Safe Resistance Training Practices:
Embarking on strength training is like starting a journey, emphasizing safety while reaping the benefits. It involves using resistance, such as weights or bands, to challenge your muscles. Think of it as a gradual ascent—begin with manageable resistance and progress at your own pace. This approach ensures you build strength without straining, making it particularly crucial for individuals with diabetes. It's like having a personalized trainer guiding you through exercises that strengthen your body safely.

3. Flexibility and Balance Activities:
Beyond strength, flexibility and balance activities add a dynamic layer to diabetes care. They're like

the agile dancers in your fitness routine, promoting overall well-being. Engaging in activities like yoga and gentle stretching improves flexibility, making everyday movements easier and reducing the risk of injuries. It's similar to incorporating a graceful rhythm into your routine, enhancing your body's ability to move with ease and stability.

4. Yoga and Gentle Stretching:
Yoga and gentle stretching emerge as diabetes-friendly heroes, promoting both physical and mental well-being. Yoga involves flowing through poses, enhancing flexibility and strength. The controlled movements and mindful breathing are like a calming breeze, reducing stress—a significant factor in diabetes management. The gentle stretches contribute to improved blood circulation, aiding in glucose transport. Incorporating yoga and stretching into your routine is like adding a daily dose of balance, flexibility, and relaxation, creating a holistic approach to diabetes care.

5. Reducing Diabetes-related Neuropathy Risk:
Engaging in strength training and flexibility activities isn't just about muscles; it's also about safeguarding against diabetes-related neuropathy. Neuropathy is like a potential roadblock, causing nerve damage.

Regular exercise, especially activities promoting flexibility and balance, reduces this risk. It's akin to maintaining smooth pathways for nerve signals, preventing complications associated with diabetes-related nerve issues.

Making Exercise a Sustainable Habit for Diabetics: A Personalized Approach

Enjoyable Activities Catered to Individual Preferences

Exercise should be like a favorite hobby, enjoyable and suited to your unique preferences. Incorporating social elements is like turning your workout into a social gathering – it adds motivation and enjoyment. Whether it's joining a fitness class or walking with a friend, the social aspect provides support. Customizing workouts to your personal enjoyment is like creating your own fitness recipe. Choose activities that bring you joy, whether it's dancing, cycling, or a serene nature walk, making exercise something you genuinely look forward to.

Incorporating Social Elements for Motivation:

Imagine exercise as a group dance; it's more enjoyable when you have company. Incorporating social elements into your routine is like inviting friends to join the dance. Whether it's a workout buddy, a class, or a team sport, the shared experience adds motivation. It's like having cheerleaders on your fitness journey, making the commitment more enjoyable and sustainable.

Customizing Workouts for Personal Enjoyment:

Turning exercise into a personalized adventure is like designing your own fitness roadmap. Customizing workouts to your preferences ensures they align with your interests and lifestyle. It's like tailoring a suit – the better it fits, the more comfortable and enjoyable the experience. Whether it's mixing different activities or focusing on one you love, making it uniquely yours ensures lasting engagement.

Setting Diabetes-specific Fitness Goals:

Making exercise a sustainable habit involves setting goals as unique as your fingerprint. Diabetes-specific fitness goals are like personalized milestones on your journey to well-being.

Gradual Progression with Blood Sugar Monitoring:

Imagine your fitness journey as a steady climb, and your blood sugar levels as checkpoints along the way. Gradual progression involves taking steps at your own pace, monitored by blood sugar levels. It's like hiking a mountain – taking breaks to ensure you're on the right path. By gradually increasing intensity and duration while monitoring blood sugar responses, you create a sustainable and safe exercise routine.

SMART Goal Setting in the Context of Diabetes:

Setting diabetes-specific goals should be like creating a roadmap with clear directions. Using SMART criteria – Specific, Measurable, Achievable, Relevant, and Time-bound – is like having a GPS for your fitness goals. For example, setting a goal to walk a specific distance within a set time frame provides clarity and ensures that your efforts align with diabetes management. These SMART goals make your exercise routine more focused, attainable, and sustainable.

In essence, making exercise sustainable for diabetics involves crafting a personalized experience. Enjoyable activities, social motivation, customized workouts, and diabetes-specific goals transform exercise into a habit that not only benefits your health but also becomes an integral and enjoyable part of your lifestyle.

Overcoming Barriers Specific to Diabetic Patients: Navigating Challenges with Precision

Time Management with Consideration for Blood Sugar Levels:

Balancing exercise with diabetes requires a masterful approach, akin to orchestrating a symphony of wellness. Strategic timing of exercise sessions is like conducting the performance – choose times when blood sugar levels are stable, avoiding extreme highs or lows. It's a dance between your body's rhythm and the clock. Balancing physical activity and meal planning is like harmonizing the notes – ensuring that your energy levels align with your activity while keeping blood sugar in check. It's about orchestrating a seamless blend that supports both your fitness goals and diabetes management.

Strategic Timing of Exercise Sessions:

Think of your exercise routine as a well-timed melody. Strategic timing involves choosing moments when your blood sugar levels are in a harmonious range. It's like selecting the right tempo – not too fast to cause a spike or too slow to risk a drop. By aligning exercise sessions with your body's natural rhythms, you optimize the impact of physical activity on your blood sugar levels.

Balancing Physical Activity and Meal Planning:

Imagine your meals as the fuel for your exercise journey. Balancing physical activity with meal planning is like creating a menu that complements your workout. It's about choosing the right nutrients at the right times to sustain energy levels and regulate blood sugar. By coordinating your meals with your exercise routine, you create a synergy that supports both your fitness aspirations and diabetes care.

Addressing Diabetes-related Health Concerns:

Overcoming barriers specific to diabetic patients involves a tailored approach, much like creating a bespoke suit. Addressing diabetes-related health concerns is like adjusting the fit – ensuring that exercises accommodate individual needs and health considerations.

Adapting Exercises for Neuropathy or Foot Health:

Navigating exercises with neuropathy or foot health concerns requires a personalized dance. Adapting exercises involves choosing movements that safeguard nerve and foot health. It's like customizing a dance routine to fit your unique style, ensuring that every step is supportive and gentle. By making modifications based on individual health concerns, you create an exercise routine that aligns with your body's needs.

Collaboration with Healthcare Professionals for Tailored Plans:

Think of healthcare professionals as your partners in this fitness journey. Collaboration involves seeking their guidance for a tailored exercise plan. It's like having a co-pilot who understands the intricacies of your health. By working closely with healthcare professionals, you ensure that your exercise routine is not just beneficial but also safe and aligned with your specific health needs.

In essence, overcoming barriers specific to diabetic patients involves a meticulous approach, considering the nuances of time management, health concerns, and collaborative planning. By addressing these challenges with precision, individuals with diabetes can create an exercise routine that not only enhances their well-being but also aligns seamlessly with their unique health requirements.

Integrating Diabetes-friendly Exercises into Daily Life

Incorporating Movement into Sedentary Settings

Making exercise a part of your daily life is like weaving wellness into the fabric of your routine. Incorporating movement into sedentary settings is akin to adding a vibrant thread to your day.

Desk Exercises and Quick Breaks

Transform your workspace into an active zone by incorporating desk exercises. Picture it as a mini dance – simple stretches, seated leg lifts, or torso twists to break up long periods of sitting. These quick breaks are like refreshing interludes in your daily symphony, preventing stiffness and enhancing blood circulation. By infusing movement into your sedentary settings, you create a dynamic flow that supports both productivity and well-being.

Integrating Activity into Work and Home Life:

Imagine your daily tasks as opportunities for a wellness dance. Integrating activity into work and home life involves choosing movement-friendly alternatives. It's like switching from an elevator to stairs or opting for a standing desk. By infusing these choices into your routine, you seamlessly blend activity into your day. It's about turning daily tasks into active moments, making wellness an integral part of your work and home experience.

Family and Community Engagement for Diabetes-friendly Activities:

Exercise becomes a shared celebration when it involves family and community. Engaging loved ones and the community in diabetes-friendly activities is like orchestrating a collective movement towards well-being.

Involving Family in Supportive Exercise Routines

Transform family time into a wellness adventure. Involving family in supportive exercise routines is like choreographing a group dance. Whether it's a family walk, a dance party, or outdoor activities, making fitness a shared experience strengthens bonds while promoting health. It's about turning exercise into a joyous occasion that everyone can participate in and benefit from.

Participating in Diabetes-focused Community Programs:

Imagine your community as a stage for collective well-being. Participating in diabetes-focused community programs is like joining a community dance. It could be group fitness classes, wellness workshops, or community walks specifically tailored for diabetes management. By engaging in these programs, you not only foster personal well-being but also contribute to a supportive community that shares similar health goals.

In summary, integrating diabetes-friendly exercises into daily life is about making wellness a seamless part of your routine. From desk exercises to active family moments and community engagement, it's a holistic approach that transforms daily life into a dance of well-being. These small, intentional steps pave the way for a healthier and more active lifestyle, making exercise an inherent and enjoyable aspect of your everyday existence.

Staying Positive with Diabetes in Mind: Taking Care of Yourself

Celebrating Diabetes Exercise Wins:

Imagine your health journey like a treasure hunt – each victory is a golden moment. Celebrating diabetes exercise wins means acknowledging the good things that happen to your body.

Noticing Sugar Level Improvements:

Picture your blood sugar levels as signs of progress. Noticing sugar level improvements is like recognizing the good changes in your journey. Whether your levels become steadier or you need less medicine, celebrating these achievements boosts your mood and shows that your efforts make a real difference.

Seeing Other Health Benefits:

Think of your well-being like a colorful artwork made by exercise. Seeing other health benefits involves noticing improvements beyond sugar control. It's like adding bright colors of better sleep, more energy, and feeling happier to your artwork. By appreciating these positive changes, you build motivation rooted in the overall good feelings that exercise brings.

Trying Different Diabetes-friendly Activities:

Keeping things interesting is like trying new foods – it makes your day more exciting. Trying different diabetes-friendly activities means adding variety to your exercise routine to make it enjoyable.

Doing Different Exercises

Think of your exercise routine as a collection of different games. Doing different exercises for diabetes involves trying various activities that help with managing your health. It's like playing different sports, lifting weights, and stretching – each one brings something unique to your routine.

Changing Exercises as Your Health Changes:

Imagine your exercise routine as a dance that adapts to your body's rhythm. Changing exercises as your health changes involves adjusting your routine when needed. It's like modifying your dance moves based on how you feel – doing more or less depending on what your body needs. Being flexible ensures that your exercise routine is always helpful and friendly to your health.

In simple terms, staying positive with diabetes in mind is about celebrating victories, noticing good changes, and making exercise fun by trying different activities. It's a happy and thankful approach that not only keeps you interested in exercising but also shows that your efforts are making your body feel good overall.

Safety Tips for Exercise

Warming Up and Cooling Down Safely:

Imagine your body as a car that needs a smooth start and a gentle stop. Warming up and cooling down safely is like the key to a smooth ride.

Importance of Checking Blood Sugar:

Think of checking your blood sugar like making sure your car has enough fuel. Before starting, it's crucial to check your blood sugar levels. It's like knowing if your car has enough gas for the journey. This helps you avoid starting with low energy and keeps you safe during exercise.

Cooling Down to Avoid Blood Sugar Drops:

After exercising, think of your body like a car engine that needs to cool down. Cooling down helps prevent sudden drops in blood sugar. It's like letting your car engine settle after a long drive. Taking a few minutes to cool down ensures a smooth transition and reduces the risk of feeling lightheaded or shaky.

Working Together with Healthcare Professionals:

Consider healthcare professionals as your travel guides on this wellness journey. Working together involves building a partnership for a safe and effective exercise plan.

Regular Check-ins and Personalized Exercise Plans

Think of check-ins with healthcare professionals like getting expert advice on your journey. Regular check-ins help them understand how you're doing. It's like having a navigator who ensures you're on the right path. Personalized exercise plans are like having a customized map for your specific needs, making your fitness journey safer and more tailored to you.

Personalizing Safety Measures Based on Individual Profiles:

Consider personalizing safety measures as having your own set of rules for the road. It involves adapting safety measures based on your unique health profile. It's like having specific guidelines for your car based on its unique features. By tailoring safety measures to your individual needs, you ensure that your exercise routine is both effective and safe.

In simple terms, staying safe during exercise with diabetes involves starting and stopping smoothly, checking your blood sugar levels like fuel, and collaborating with healthcare professionals as your trusted guides. It's a careful and personalized approach that makes your fitness journey both enjoyable and secure.

Chapter 4

Lifestyle Adjustments - Stress Management Techniques

In Chapter 4, we delve into effective stress management techniques. From mindfulness practices to relaxation exercises, this chapter provides a comprehensive guide to help readers navigate and alleviate the impact of stress on their well-being.

Understanding the link between stress and Blood Sugar Levels

When we're stressed, our bodies react in a way that can influence our blood sugar levels. Imagine your body as a finely tuned orchestra, with each instrument playing a crucial role. When stress comes into play, it's like the conductor signaling a change in the music.

Stress prompts the release of certain hormones, such as cortisol and adrenaline, which are like messengers telling your body to prepare for action. These messengers can also lead to an increase in blood sugar. It's a bit like putting more fuel into a car to rev up the engine – your body is getting ready for a burst of energy.

Now, the tricky part is that for people with diabetes, this natural response can cause a challenge. The extra sugar released into the bloodstream might not be managed effectively by insulin, the hormone responsible for regulating blood sugar. It's as if the usual traffic cop (insulin) gets a bit overwhelmed with all the extra vehicles (sugar) on the road.

Consistent high levels of blood sugar can lead to various health issues, so understanding and managing this link is crucial. Picture it as finding the right balance in our orchestra – not too fast, not too slow.

Effectively managing stress becomes a key player in this symphony. Simple practices like taking a few deep breaths, going for a walk, or practicing mindfulness can be powerful tools. It's like giving the orchestra a moment to pause, regroup, and play harmoniously again.

In essence, grasping the link between stress and blood sugar is about recognizing the interconnected dance of our body's responses. By taking mindful steps to manage stress, we can help keep the orchestra – our body – in tune and promote overall well-being, especially for those managing diabetes.

Tips on managing stress levels

Managing stress is like taking care of a garden – it requires a bit of attention and some nurturing. In our busy lives, stress can sneak up on us, but with a few simple strategies, we can cultivate a sense of calm.

1. Take a Breath: One of the easiest and most effective ways to dial down stress is to take deep breaths. Imagine you're smelling a flower – breathe in slowly through your nose, hold it for a moment, and then exhale gently. It's like giving your mind and body a little reset button.

2. Move Your Body: Physical activity isn't just good for your muscles; it's a fantastic stress-buster too. You don't need to run a marathon – a short walk, some stretching, or even dancing around your living room can work wonders. It's like telling your body, "Hey, let's shake off this stress together!"

3. Break Tasks into Bits: When faced with a mountain of tasks, it can feel overwhelming. Break things into smaller, manageable bits. It's like eating a slice of cake rather than the whole thing – one piece at a time is much more doable.

4. Talk It Out: Sharing your thoughts and feelings with someone you trust is like letting out a balloon filled with stress. It could be a friend, a family member, or even a pet. Expressing what's on your mind can make the load feel lighter.

5. Create a Happy List: Make a list of things that make you happy or bring a smile to your face. It could be as simple as enjoying a cup of tea, listening to your favorite song, or spending time with a loved one. When stress creeps in, turn to your happy list for a boost.

6. Practice Mindfulness: This might sound fancy, but it's like giving your brain a mini-vacation. Mindfulness is about being in the present moment. You can start with short sessions – just focus on your breath or the sights and sounds around you. It's a bit like pressing pause on life's fast-forward button.

Remember, managing stress is a journey, not a race. These simple tips are like tools in your stress-busting toolbox. Experiment with them, find what works best for you, and gradually weave them into your daily routine. Like tending to a garden, a little care for yourself can lead to a more peaceful and balanced life.

Chapter 5

Natural Remedies

Chapter 5 delves into the realm of natural remedies, offering a tapestry of alternative approaches to enhance health and well-being. From herbal remedies to ancient practices, this chapter explores the therapeutic potential of nature's offerings, inviting readers to consider a holistic approach to nurturing their health.

Holistic Approaches to Diabetes Management

When it comes to managing diabetes holistically, it's not just about counting carbs or hitting the gym. Imagine your health as a puzzle, and each piece contributes to the bigger picture of well-being.

1. Mind-Body Practices:
   Incorporating mind-body practices like mindfulness and relaxation techniques is like giving your mind a spa day. These practices not only reduce stress but also have a positive impact on

71

blood sugar levels. Think of it as creating a serene oasis within, where the ripples of calmness extend to your overall health.

2. Quality Sleep:

Picture your body as a restoration hub. Adequate sleep is like the nightly maintenance session, ensuring all systems are in top-notch condition. It's not just about the hours; it's about the quality of sleep. Establishing a consistent sleep routine can be a powerful tool in diabetes management, promoting better blood sugar control and overall vitality.

3. Social Connections:

Imagine your support system as the wind beneath your wings. Strong social connections are like a safety net, providing emotional support and encouragement. Whether through friends, family, or community groups, these connections act as pillars in your diabetes journey. Sharing experiences and victories creates a sense of community that fosters well-being.

4. Creative Outlets:

Engaging in creative pursuits is like adding color to your diabetes management canvas. Whether it's art, music, or writing, these outlets provide a means of expression and stress relief. They're not just hobbies; they are therapeutic tools that contribute to emotional balance and resilience.

5. Holistic Therapies:
   Exploring holistic therapies like acupuncture or massage is like offering your body alternative pathways to wellness. These therapies aim to balance energy and promote overall harmony. While not substitutes for traditional medical approaches, they can complement your diabetes management plan, adding diverse layers to your health strategy.

6. Goal Setting and Tracking:
   Setting realistic goals and tracking progress is like creating a roadmap for success. It's not about aiming for perfection but establishing achievable milestones. Regularly assessing and adjusting your goals, in collaboration with your healthcare team, ensures you stay on course and maintain a sense of control over your diabetes management journey.

In embracing a holistic approach to diabetes management, the focus extends beyond traditional pillars like diet and exercise. It's about nurturing a symphony of elements that contribute to your overall well-being. By recognizing the interconnected nature of these practices, you empower yourself to create a vibrant, balanced life with diabetes.

Herbal Supplements

Managing diabetes involves a multifaceted strategy, and herbal supplements have emerged as potential allies in this journey. These natural remedies, derived from plants and herbs, offer a complementary avenue alongside conventional treatments. In this exploration, we will delve into various herbal supplements, their potential benefits, and how to incorporate them into your diabetes management plan.

1. Bitter Melon (Momordica charantia):
Benefits: Bitter melon, resembling a bumpy cucumber, contains compounds that may help lower blood sugar levels. It's like a natural sugar regulator in your garden of health. Consuming bitter melon, whether in its raw form, as a juice, or in supplement

capsules, has been associated with improved glucose tolerance.

How to Use: Incorporate bitter melon into your diet by stir-frying, juicing, or blending it into smoothies. For those preferring supplements, capsules are available, but consulting with a healthcare professional before adding them to your routine is advisable.

2. Fenugreek (Trigonella foenum-graecum):

Benefits: Fenugreek seeds, reminiscent of small golden nuggets, contain soluble fiber and compounds that may aid in managing blood sugar levels. Think of fenugreek as a gentle assistant, supporting your body in its efforts to balance glucose.

How to Use: Soak fenugreek seeds overnight and consume them in the morning. They can also be ground into a powder and added to dishes or taken in capsule form. As with any supplement, moderation and consultation with a healthcare provider are crucial.

3. Cinnamon (Cinnamomum verum):

Benefits: Beyond its aromatic allure, cinnamon holds potential benefits for those with diabetes. It may improve insulin sensitivity, acting like a friendly guide for insulin to do its job effectively.

How to Use: Sprinkle cinnamon on your morning oatmeal, yogurt, or incorporate it into your favorite recipes. Cinnamon supplements are also available, but moderation and regular monitoring of blood sugar levels are essential.

4. Aloe Vera:

Benefits: Aloe vera, known for its soothing properties, may also contribute to diabetes management. It contains compounds that could enhance insulin sensitivity, acting as a natural support system.

How to Use: Harvest the gel from fresh aloe vera leaves and add it to smoothies or consume it directly. Aloe vera supplements are available, but it's advisable to consult with a healthcare professional due to potential interactions with medications.

5. Ginseng:

Benefits: Ginseng, with its forked root resembling the limbs of a person, has been studied for its potential to improve blood sugar control. It's like a wise companion, aiding your body in maintaining balance.

How to Use: Ginseng can be consumed as a tea or taken in supplement form. However, due to potential interactions and varied effects, it's crucial to consult with a healthcare provider before incorporating ginseng into your routine.

6. Turmeric (Curcuma longa):
Benefits: Turmeric, with its vibrant golden hue, contains curcumin, known for its anti-inflammatory properties. It may have potential benefits in managing diabetes by reducing inflammation.

How to Use: Incorporate turmeric into your cooking, make golden milk with turmeric and warm milk, or consider turmeric supplements after consulting with a healthcare professional.

7. Gymnema Sylvestre:
Benefits: Gymnema sylvestre, known as the "sugar destroyer," may help reduce sugar

absorption in the intestines and enhance insulin function.

How to Use: Gymnema supplements are available, but it's crucial to consult with a healthcare provider for proper dosage and potential interactions.

8. Neem (Azadirachta indica):
Benefits: Neem, often called the "wonder leaf," has compounds that may help lower blood sugar levels and enhance insulin sensitivity.

How to Use: Neem leaves can be consumed as tea or added to dishes. Neem supplements are also available, but consultation with a healthcare professional is recommended.

9. Acai Berry:
Benefits: Acai berries, resembling small, dark purple gems, are rich in antioxidants and fiber. While research on their direct impact on blood sugar is limited, their overall nutritional profile may support general well-being.

How to Use: Incorporate acai berries into smoothies, bowls, or snacks. Acai supplements are also available, but it's essential to consult with a healthcare professional for guidance.

10. Apple Cider Vinegar:
  Benefits: Apple cider vinegar, a pantry staple, may have potential benefits in improving insulin sensitivity and lowering blood sugar levels after meals.

  How to Use: Dilute a small amount of apple cider vinegar in water and consume before meals. It can also be used in salad dressings. However, moderation is key, and it's advisable to consult with a healthcare provider, especially for those with existing digestive issues.

Incorporating Herbal Supplements Safely:
  - Consult with a healthcare professional before adding any herbal supplement to your routine.
  - Monitor blood sugar levels regularly to assess the impact of supplements.
  - Be mindful of potential interactions between herbal supplements and medications.
  - Emphasize moderation, as excessive intake of even natural substances may have adverse effects.

- Remember that herbal supplements should complement, not replace, conventional diabetes management approaches.

While herbal supplements offer potential benefits, they are not a one-size-fits-all solution. Individual responses may vary, and personalized guidance from healthcare providers is paramount. In the garden of diabetes management, these herbal allies can be cultivated wisely, contributing to a holistic approach that considers the intricate balance of nature and health.

Chapter 6

Recipes for a Balanced Life

Diabetes-Friendly Meal Plans

Meal Plan 1: Mediterranean Flavors

***Breakfast*:**
  - Greek yogurt parfait with layers of mixed berries, a drizzle of honey, and a sprinkle of almonds.
  - Whole-grain toast with olive tapenade.

Lunch:
  - Grilled chicken or chickpea salad with mixed greens, cherry tomatoes, cucumber, feta cheese, and a lemon vinaigrette.
  - Quinoa or bulgur on the side.

Snack:
  - Hummus with carrot and cucumber sticks.

Dinner:
  - Baked white fish with a Mediterranean salsa (tomatoes, olives, capers).

- Roasted sweet potatoes and asparagus.

Snack (if needed):
- Handful of mixed nuts.

Meal Plan 2: Asian Fusion

Breakfast:
- Vegetable and tofu stir-fry with a light soy sauce.
- Brown rice on the side.

Lunch:
- Sushi bowl with cauliflower rice, avocado, cucumber, and sashimi-grade fish or tofu.
- Miso soup.

Snack:
- Edamame with a sprinkle of sea salt.

Dinner:
- Chicken or tofu curry with broccoli and bell peppers.
- Quinoa or basmati rice.

Snack (if needed):
- Sliced mango with a squeeze of lime.

Meal Plan 3: Classic Comfort

Breakfast:
- Oatmeal made with rolled oats, almond milk, and topped with sliced bananas and a sprinkle of cinnamon.
- Scrambled eggs or tofu.

Lunch:
- Turkey or veggie chili with kidney beans, tomatoes, and bell peppers.
- Whole-grain crackers on the side.

Snack:
- Cottage cheese with pineapple chunks.

Dinner:
- Grilled salmon or portobello mushrooms.
- Quinoa or wild rice.
- Steamed green beans.

Snack (if needed):
- Apple slices with almond butter.

Meal Plan 4: Tex-Mex Twist

Breakfast:

- Breakfast burrito with scrambled eggs or tofu, black beans, salsa, and whole-grain tortilla.
- Sliced avocado on the side.

Lunch:
- Chicken or black bean salad bowl with lettuce, tomatoes, corn, and a lime-cilantro dressing.
- Brown rice.

Snack:
- Guacamole with whole-grain tortilla chips.

Dinner:
- Grilled shrimp or vegetable fajitas with peppers and onions.
- Quinoa or whole-grain tortillas.

Snack (if needed):
- Mixed fruit salsa with cinnamon tortilla chips.

Meal Plan 5: Quick and Easy

Breakfast:
- Smoothie with spinach, banana, almond milk, and a scoop of protein powder.
- Whole-grain toast with peanut butter.

Lunch:
  - Turkey or veggie wrap with whole-grain tortilla, lettuce, tomato, and a smear of hummus.
  - Carrot sticks on the side.

Snack:
  - String cheese with cherry tomatoes.

Dinner:
  - Baked chicken or tofu with lemon and herbs.
  - Quinoa or couscous.
  - Steamed broccoli.

Snack (if needed):
  - Mixed nuts or seeds.

Meal Plan 6: Fresh and Light

Breakfast:
  - Fruit salad with a dollop of Greek yogurt.
  - Whole-grain English muffin with cream cheese.

Lunch:
  - Shrimp or avocado salad with mixed greens, mango, and a citrus vinaigrette.
  - Brown rice or quinoa.

Snack:
- Cottage cheese with sliced strawberries.

Dinner:
- Grilled fish tacos with slaw and avocado.
- Cauliflower rice.

Snack (if needed):
- Sliced cucumber with tzatziki.

Meal Plan 7: Hearty and Filling

Breakfast:
- Scrambled eggs with sautéed spinach and whole-grain toast.
- Berries on the side.

Lunch:
- Lentil soup with a side of whole-grain crackers.
- Mixed green salad with a light vinaigrette.

Snack:
- Greek yogurt with a sprinkle of granola.

Dinner:
- Baked chicken or tempeh with rosemary and sweet potatoes.

- Steamed green beans.

Snack (if needed):
  - Apple slices with a small piece of cheese.

Considerations:
  - Adjust portion sizes based on individual needs.
  - Be mindful of carbohydrate intake and distribute it evenly throughout the day.
  - Stay hydrated with water or herbal teas.
  - Consult with healthcare professionals or dietitians for personalized guidance.

These meal plans offer a variety of flavors and ingredients, providing options for different tastes and preferences. As always, it's important to tailor these plans to individual health needs and consult with healthcare professionals for personalized guidance on managing diabetes through diet.

Chapter 7

Medication and Treatment Options

Overview of Diabetes Medications

Managing diabetes often involves medications to help control blood sugar levels. There are various classes of medications, each with its unique mechanisms of action. It's important to note that the choice of medication depends on individual factors such as the type of diabetes, overall health, and specific needs. Here's an overview of common diabetes medications:

1. Metformin:
   - How it works: Decreases glucose production by the liver and improves insulin sensitivity.
   - Considerations: Typically a first-line treatment for type 2 diabetes. May cause gastrointestinal side effects.

2. Sulfonylureas (e.g., Glipizide, Glimepiride):

- How they work: Stimulate the pancreas to release more insulin.
- Considerations: Can cause low blood sugar (hypoglycemia) and may be associated with weight gain.

3. Meglitinides (e.g., Repaglinide, Nateglinide):
- How they work: Stimulate insulin release from the pancreas, but their action is shorter-lived compared to sulfonylureas.
- Considerations: Taken before meals and may cause hypoglycemia.

4. Thiazolidinediones (e.g., Pioglitazone, Rosiglitazone):
- How they work: Improve insulin sensitivity in cells and decrease glucose production in the liver.
- Considerations: May cause weight gain and fluid retention. Regular monitoring for potential side effects is essential.

5. Dipeptidyl Peptidase-4 (DPP-4) Inhibitors (e.g., Sitagliptin, Saxagliptin):
- How they work: Increase insulin release and decrease glucagon production after meals.
- Considerations: Generally well-tolerated but may cause joint pain.

6. Sodium-Glucose Cotransporter-2 (SGLT2) Inhibitors (e.g., Canagliflozin, Empagliflozin):

- How they work: Block the reabsorption of glucose by the kidneys, leading to increased glucose excretion in urine.
- Considerations: Can lower blood pressure and may increase the risk of urinary tract infections.

7. Insulin:

- How it works: Replaces or supplements the body's insulin, helping to regulate blood sugar.
- Considerations: Different types of insulin with various onset and duration times. Administered via injections or insulin pumps.

8. GLP-1 Receptor Agonists (e.g., Liraglutide, Dulaglutide):

- How they work: Increase insulin release, reduce glucagon production, and slow down digestion, leading to lower blood sugar levels.
- Considerations: May cause weight loss and have cardiovascular benefits.

9. Combination Medications:

- How they work: Provide the benefits of multiple medications in one convenient form.

- Considerations: Prescribed based on individual needs and may improve medication adherence.

It's crucial for individuals with diabetes to work closely with healthcare professionals to determine the most suitable medication or combination of medications. Regular monitoring, lifestyle adjustments, and medication adherence are key components of effective diabetes management. As medical advancements continue, new medications and treatment options may become available to further enhance diabetes care.

Emerging Treatment Approaches

1. Precision Medicine:
- Significance: Tailoring diabetes treatments based on an individual's genetic, environmental, and lifestyle factors.

2. Artificial Pancreas Systems:
- Significance: Integrating continuous glucose monitoring with insulin delivery in a closed-loop system for real-time adjustments.

3. GLP-1/GIP Receptor Dual Agonists:

- Significance: Stimulating both GLP-1 and GIP receptors to target multiple pathways involved in glucose regulation.

4. Cell Replacement Therapy:

- Significance: Exploring the replacement of damaged or dysfunctional pancreatic cells with healthy cells, including beta-cell transplantation.

5. Stem Cell Therapy:

- Significance: Investigating the potential of stem cells to differentiate into insulin-producing cells, offering a regenerative approach.

Chapter 8

Managing Blood Sugar Spikes and Hypoglycemia

Chapter 8 delves into the essential topic of "Managing Blood Sugar Spikes," providing practical insights for individuals navigating diabetes. Understanding and controlling blood sugar levels is crucial for overall well-being. This chapter explores the factors contributing to spikes, including diet, physical activity, and stress. Readers will discover effective strategies to prevent and address sudden increases in blood sugar, empowering them to make informed lifestyle choices. From dietary modifications to mindful practices, the chapter offers a comprehensive guide to maintaining stable blood sugar levels, enhancing daily life for those managing diabetes. Join this exploration for actionable tips towards achieving better blood sugar management.

Recognizing and Understanding Spikes

Understanding spikes in blood sugar is really important for people with diabetes. Imagine your blood sugar levels like a roller coaster – you want a smooth ride, not sudden ups and downs. A spike happens when the roller coaster goes up too fast.

Now, why do these spikes happen? One big reason is the food we eat. If you have lots of sugary or high-carb foods, it's like putting extra fuel in the roller coaster, making it go up quickly. Lack of exercise is like having a slow roller coaster – it doesn't burn the fuel well, causing sugar to stay high.

Stress is another player in this game. When stress hits, it's like pressing a button that makes the roller coaster go up suddenly. Our body releases special chemicals, and they tell the roller coaster to speed up.

How do you know if there's a spike? Watch out for signs like feeling very thirsty, tired, or having blurry vision. Testing your blood sugar helps catch these spikes early. It's like having a superpower to see what's happening on the roller coaster.

Continuous glucose monitoring (CGM) is like having a superhero sidekick. It shows your sugar levels in real-time, helping you understand how food, exercise, and stress affect your roller coaster.

Knowing is half the battle. Once you understand spikes, you can make smart choices. Eat balanced meals – not too much fuel for the roller coaster. Move around to keep the roller coaster on track. And when stress tries to press that button, use calming tricks like deep breaths.

Understanding spikes is like having a map for your blood sugar journey. It puts you in control, helping you enjoy a smoother ride on the roller coaster of diabetes.

Immediate Action Tips:

1. Cinnamon Trick:
   - Sprinkle a bit of cinnamon on your meals; it may help regulate blood sugar.

2. Green Tea Boost:
   - Sip on green tea; it contains antioxidants that could aid in sugar control.

   - Mix chia seeds in water; they form a gel that slows sugar absorption.

4. Apple Cider Vinegar Shot:
   - Take a small shot of diluted apple cider vinegar; some find it helps manage blood sugar.

5. Fiber Fix:
   - Grab a fiber-rich snack, like raw veggies or berries, to stabilize sugar levels.

6. Lemon Water Refresh:
   - Drink water with a squeeze of lemon; hydration can support glucose balance.

7. Berries Bonanza:
   - Enjoy a handful of berries; they offer natural sweetness without spiking sugar.

8. Fenugreek Magic:
   - Try fenugreek seeds; they may assist in controlling blood sugar levels.

9. Yogurt Soothe:
- Opt for plain yogurt; its probiotics might have positive effects on sugar.

10. Spice it Up with Turmeric:
- Add turmeric to your meals; its active compound could aid in sugar regulation.

The Don'ts following a spike

What Not to Do After a Blood Sugar Spike:

1. Avoid Sugary Snacks:
- Resist the urge to grab sugary treats; they can make the spike worse.

2. Say No to Large Meals:
- Skip large, high-carb meals; they can keep your sugar levels high.

3. Hold Off on Strenuous Exercise:
- Avoid intense workouts immediately; it might raise your blood sugar more.

4. Don't Stress Out:
- Try not to stress; it can make blood sugar harder to control.

5. Say No to Soda:
   - Don't choose sugary drinks; they can quickly spike your blood sugar.

6. Don't Ignore Hydration:
   - Don't forget to drink water; staying hydrated helps flush out excess sugar.

Managing Low Blood Sugar

Recognizing Hypoglycemia

Hypoglycemia, or low blood sugar, is important to recognize for those managing diabetes. Here are signs to watch for:

1. Feeling Shaky:
   - Trembling hands or feeling shaky can be an early sign of low blood sugar.

2. Sweating:
   - Experiencing sudden sweats, especially if they're cold or clammy.

3. Dizziness:

- Feeling lightheaded or dizzy, as if you might faint.

4. Irritability:
   - Becoming easily irritated, anxious, or unusually moody.

5. Weakness:
   - Generalized weakness or fatigue can indicate low blood sugar.

6. Confusion:
   - Difficulty concentrating or confusion may arise.

7. Hunger:
   - Suddenly feeling very hungry, even if you've recently eaten.

8. Blurred Vision:
   - Vision changes or blurriness can occur during hypoglycemia.

9. Headache:
   - Developing a headache that is not usual for you.

10. Nausea:
    - Feeling nauseous or having an upset stomach.

It's essential to treat hypoglycemia promptly. Consuming a quick source of glucose, like fruit juice, candy, or glucose tablets, can help raise blood sugar.

Immediate Response Measures

1. Consume Fast-Acting Carbs:
   - Eat or drink a quick source of glucose, such as fruit juice, a glucose gel, or several pieces of candy.

2. Recheck Blood Sugar:
   - Test your blood sugar 15 minutes after consuming glucose to ensure it's rising.

3. Follow with a Snack:
   - Have a small, balanced snack containing protein and carbohydrates to sustain blood sugar levels.

4. Rest:
   - Rest for a short period to allow your body to recover.

5. Inform Others:
   - Let someone know about your hypoglycemia episode, especially if you need assistance.

6. Avoid Overeating:
   - While it's essential to consume glucose, avoid overeating to prevent a subsequent blood sugar spike.

7. Monitor Symptoms:
   - Keep an eye on your symptoms to ensure they improve. If not, seek medical assistance.

8. Stay Hydrated
   - Drink water to stay hydrated, as dehydration can worsen symptoms.

9. Avoid Driving:
   - Refrain from driving until you're sure your blood sugar is stable.

10. Medical Assistance if Needed:
    - If symptoms persist, become severe, or you're unable to treat yourself, seek immediate medical help.

Long-term Strategies for Prevention

Things to Avoid to Prevent Low Sugar:

1. Don't Forget Meals:
   - Always eat your meals and snacks to keep your sugar levels steady.

2. Avoid Too Much Alcohol:
   - If you drink, don't overdo it, and have some food with it to avoid low sugar.

3. Go Easy on Intense Exercise:
   - Don't do super hard exercise without having a little snack first.

4. Keep Carbs Consistent:
   - Try to eat the same amount of carb-rich foods each meal to avoid sugar ups and downs.

5. No DIY Medication Changes:
   - Don't change your medicine without talking to your doctor first.

6. Listen to Symptoms:
   - If you feel shaky or strange, don't ignore it. Treat it right away.

7. Not Only Quick Sugars:
   - While quick sugar helps, don't rely only on candies. Aim for good meals too.

8. Stay Hydrated:
   - Don't forget to drink water. Dehydration can mess with your sugar.

Things to Do to Prevent Low Sugar:

1. Check Sugar Regularly:
   - Keep an eye on your sugar levels to know what's happening.

2. Mix Up Your Meals:
   - Eat a mix of foods – some carbs, some protein, and healthy fats in your meals.

3. Same Time, Same Meal:
   - Try to eat meals and snacks at the same time every day.

4. Healthy Snacks Rule:
   - Have healthy snacks between meals to keep your sugar steady.

5. Move Your Body:
   - Do some exercise regularly. It helps your body handle sugar better.

6. Take Your Meds Right:
   - Take your medicine just like your doctor says. If something feels off, tell them.

7. Let Others Know:
   - Tell people close to you about signs of low sugar and what to do. It's good to have backup.

8. Learn About Sugar:
   - Keep learning about low sugar and how to deal with it. Knowledge is your superpower.

9. Drink Water:
   - Don't forget to drink water. It's important for your body, especially with diabetes.

10. Ask Your Doctor:
   - If you have questions or worries, ask your doctor. They're there to help you.

Keeping things simple and consistent helps you manage your sugar levels better. These steps can be like your daily checklist to stay on track.

Chapter 9

Monitoring Blood Sugar Levels

Chapter 9 delves into the critical aspect of "Monitoring Blood Sugar Levels," an indispensable practice for effective diabetes management. This chapter aims to empower individuals with practical insights into the significance of regular monitoring, the tools available, and how to interpret the results. Understanding your blood sugar levels is akin to having a compass in the journey of diabetes, guiding you towards informed decisions on lifestyle, medication, and overall well-being. Join us in exploring the essential role of monitoring in maintaining stability, making proactive adjustments, and achieving long-term success in the management of diabetes.

Best Times to Check Blood Sugar

1. When You Wake Up:

- Check your sugar in the morning before eating anything.

2. Before Meals:
   - Before lunch and dinner, so you know where your sugar starts.

3. Two Hours After Meals:
   - Check about two hours after meals to see how your body handles what you ate.

4. Before Bed:
   - Just before going to bed, to understand your sugar level before sleeping.

5. If You Feel Off:
   - Anytime you feel shaky or strange, check your sugar to catch any issues.

6. During Exercise:
   - If you're exercising, check to make sure your sugar is okay during and after.

7. When Trying Something New:
   - If you're trying new foods or activities, check to understand how they affect your sugar.

Interpreting Results

1. Fasting Blood Sugar (Morning):
- Normal Range: 70-130 mg/dL
- Interpretation: A good level before eating in the morning.

2. Before Meals:
- Normal Range: 70-130 mg/dL
- Interpretation: Ideal sugar level before eating.

3. Two Hours After Meals:
- Normal Range: Less than 180 mg/dL
- Interpretation: Checking how your body handles food; it should be lower than this after meals.

4. Before Bed:
- Normal Range: 100-140 mg/dL
- Interpretation: A good level before sleeping.

5. When You Feel Off:
- Normal Range: Varies
- Interpretation: Compare to your usual levels; low readings might mean you need a snack.

6. During Exercise:

- Normal Range: Varies
- Interpretation: Check if your sugar is stable during and after exercise.

7. Trying Something New:

- Interpretation: Compare to your usual readings; observe how new foods or activities affect your sugar.

Important Notes:
- Too Low (Hypoglycemia): Below 70 mg/dL – Eat or drink something with quick sugar.
- Too High (Hyperglycemia): Above 180 mg/dL (two hours after meals) – Consult your healthcare provider; it might indicate a need for adjustments.

Understanding these numbers helps you make decisions about food, medication, and lifestyle to keep your sugar in a healthy range. Always discuss your results with your healthcare provider for personalized guidance.

Using Data for Informed Decision-Making

1. Understanding Trends:
- Look at patterns over time to see how your sugar behaves at different moments.

2. Mealtime Adjustments:
- If your sugar is often high after meals, you might adjust what and how much you eat.

3. Medication Guidance:
- Share your data with your healthcare provider. It helps them adjust your medicine if needed.

4. Spotting Triggers:
- Check if certain foods or activities consistently affect your sugar levels.

5. Preventing Lows:
- If your sugar drops often, use the data to plan snacks and prevent hypoglycemia.

6. Setting Goals:

- Use your numbers to set realistic goals for your sugar levels with the help of your healthcare team.

7. Improving Habits:
   - Identify areas for improvement, like more exercise or changes in meals, based on your data.

8. Celebrating Success:
   - Celebrate when you see positive changes. It's a sign your efforts are paying off.

9. Effective Communication:
   - Discuss your data with your healthcare team openly. It helps them guide you better.

10. Empowering Yourself:
    - By understanding your data, you become an active participant in managing your diabetes.

Chapter 10

Thriving with Diabetes

Welcome to the final chapter of your journey, where we focus on not just managing but thriving with diabetes. In these pages, we'll explore how your efforts, dedication, and the positive changes you've made can lead to a life filled with well-being. It's not just about coping; it's about embracing a vibrant, healthy, and fulfilling life while living with diabetes. Let's celebrate your successes and discover the keys to not just surviving, but truly thriving with diabetes. This chapter is your roadmap to a future filled with vitality, joy, and continued well-being.

Success Stories

Success Story 1: Emma's Empowering Journey

Meet Emma, whose determination turned her diabetes journey into a story of triumph. Faced with a diabetes diagnosis, Emma embraced a lifestyle overhaul. She adopted a wholesome diet rich in fruits, vegetables, and whole grains while bidding farewell to processed foods. Regular walks and enjoyable workouts became a part of her routine.

Through consistent effort and a focus on weight management, Emma witnessed a remarkable shift. Her blood sugar levels stabilized, and under medical supervision, she gradually reduced her reliance on diabetes medications. Emma's success not only lies in achieving remission but in sustaining it through mindful living, showing that positive choices can rewrite the script of diabetes.

Success Story 2: James' Journey to Wellness

James, diagnosed with diabetes, embarked on a journey towards remission with unwavering commitment. He embraced a tailored exercise routine, blending aerobic activities and strength training. James discovered the power of personalized nutrition, prioritizing nutrient-dense foods and controlling portion sizes.

As James shed excess weight, the positive impact on his diabetes management became evident. Regular check-ins with healthcare professionals guided his progress. With time, James experienced a reduction in blood sugar levels, enabling a gradual adjustment of his medication. His story illustrates how the synergy of exercise, nutrition, and medical guidance can pave the way to diabetes remission and a healthier, thriving life.

Embracing a Positive Mindset

Embracing a positive mindset is like opening a door to a brighter perspective on your diabetes journey. It involves cultivating an optimistic outlook, focusing on what you can control, and finding strength in challenges. By shifting your mindset, you empower yourself to face the realities of diabetes with resilience and hope.

Key Aspects of Embracing a Positive Mindset:

1. Gratitude: Acknowledge the positive aspects of your life and health. Expressing gratitude for the good moments, no matter how small, can foster a positive mindset.

2. Focus on Solutions: Instead of dwelling on challenges, shift your focus to finding solutions.

Approach each hurdle as an opportunity for growth and learning.

3. Self-Compassion: Be kind to yourself. Understand that managing diabetes is a journey, and setbacks are a natural part of it. Treat yourself with the same kindness you would offer a friend.

4. Mindful Living: Practice mindfulness to stay present and appreciate each moment. Mindful living allows you to navigate stressors with a calm and collected mindset.

5. Set Realistic Goals: Establish achievable goals that align with your well-being. Celebrate small victories, and use them as stepping stones toward larger achievements.

6. Surround Yourself with Support: Seek support from friends, family, or a diabetes community. Building a network of encouragement can uplift your spirits during challenging times.

7. Positive Affirmations: Incorporate positive affirmations into your daily routine. Remind yourself of your strengths, capabilities, and the progress you've made.

Embracing a positive mindset doesn't mean ignoring difficulties but facing them with an attitude of resilience and hope. By fostering positivity, you empower yourself to navigate the complexities of diabetes with strength, allowing room for growth, self-discovery, and a more fulfilling life.

Planning for Long-Term Wellness, Preventing Setbacks and Maintaining Remission

Planning for Long-Term Wellness: Navigating a Future of Health

Planning for long-term wellness is like charting a course for a journey of continued health and happiness. It involves thoughtful strategies, realistic goals, and a commitment to sustaining the positive changes that have led to remission. By adopting a proactive approach, you set the stage for a future filled with well-being and minimized setbacks.

Key Aspects of Planning for Long-Term Wellness:

1. Consistent Monitoring:
   - Regularly check your blood sugar levels to stay informed about your body's responses.
   - Monitoring provides valuable insights, allowing for timely adjustments to your lifestyle plan.

2. Nutrition as a Foundation:
   - Maintain a balanced and nutritious diet with a focus on whole foods.
   - Make mindful choices, keeping portion control and the glycemic index in mind.

3. Stay Active:
   - Continue engaging in regular physical activity that suits your preferences and health status.
   - Exercise helps maintain weight, improves insulin sensitivity, and contributes to overall well-being.

4. Weight Management:
   - Strive to maintain a healthy weight through sustainable habits.
   - Weight management is closely linked to diabetes control and long-term wellness.

5. Stress Reduction:
   - Practice stress-reducing activities such as mindfulness, meditation, or hobbies.

- Managing stress is crucial for preventing setbacks and supporting overall health.

6. Regular Healthcare Check-ups:
   - Schedule regular check-ups with healthcare professionals to monitor your overall health.
   - Collaborate with your healthcare team for ongoing guidance and adjustments to your wellness plan.

Preventing Setbacks and Maintaining Remission: Nurturing Your Success

Preventing setbacks is like safeguarding the progress you've made on your wellness journey. It involves staying vigilant, adapting to changes, and addressing challenges promptly to sustain remission.

Strategies for Preventing Setbacks and Maintaining Remission:

1. Adapt to Life Changes:
   - Be flexible in adjusting your wellness plan to accommodate life changes.
   - Changes in routine, stressors, or health conditions may require tweaks to your strategy.

2. Continuous Education:
   - Stay informed about diabetes management through ongoing education.
   - Knowledge empowers you to make informed decisions and respond effectively to potential challenges.

3. Support System:
   - Maintain connections with a supportive network of friends, family, or a diabetes community.
   - A strong support system provides encouragement during both triumphs and setbacks.

4. Regular Reflective Practices:
   - Periodically reflect on your journey, celebrating achievements and identifying areas for improvement.
   - Reflective practices help you stay motivated and make necessary adjustments.

5. Anticipate and Manage Stress:
   - Proactively address stressors, recognizing their impact on overall well-being.
   - Develop coping mechanisms and seek support when needed to manage stress effectively.

Planning for long-term wellness and preventing setbacks is a continuous process. It involves a blend of consistency, adaptability, and a positive mindset. By embracing these principles, you pave the way for a future marked by sustained well-being and the ongoing joy of thriving with diabetes.

Conclusion: A Journey of Triumph and Well-Being

In closing, your journey with diabetes is a tale of triumph and well-being. By embracing positive changes, managing setbacks, and nurturing a hopeful mindset, you've paved the way for a future filled with health and happiness. Remember, this journey is ongoing, and your commitment to long-term wellness is the key. Continue monitoring, staying active, and cherishing the victories, big and small. As you navigate the path ahead, let your story inspire others. If you found this guide helpful, please consider sharing your experience through a review and good rating. Your words may light the way for someone embarking on their own journey.

Printed in Great Britain
by Amazon